144 HERBAL REMEDIES FOR NATURAL HEALING

Disclaimer

The information supplied in this book by Eliyah Mashiach is for general informational purposes only.

UNDER NO CIRCUMSTANCES SHALL WE BE LIABLE TO YOU FOR ANY LOSS OR DAMAGE OF ANY KIND INCURRED AS A RESULT OF YOUR USE OF THE SITE, DEPENDENCE ON ANY INFORMATION CONTAINED ON THIS SITE, OR USE OF ANY INFORMATION CONTAINED IN THIS SITE OR BOOK. USING THE INFORMATION SUPPLIED IS SOLELY AT YOUR OWN RISK.

Table of Contents

INTRODUCTION   1

- **HERPES**   3
- **ECZEMA**   12
- **ASTHMA**   21
- **THE COMMON FLU**   26
- **GLAUCOMA**   41
- **CATARACT**   52
- **EAR ACHE**   63
- **EAR INFECTION**   74
- **DEPRESSION**   86
- **MIGRAINE**   96
- **GINGIVITIS**   107
- **CANKER SORES**   120

CONCLUSION   133

NOTES PAGES   135

Introduction

Greetings everyone!!! I am Eliyah Mashiach a Natural Herbalist. In this book, I will be sharing with you all 144 herbal remedies for 12 of the most common illnesses that you have to deal with every day. This is a simple handy book to keep at home that is of great value and benefit to the entire family as well as your neighbors. I truly hope that you find each remedy beneficial.

Pleasant reading!

HERPES

Remedy 1 Echinacea and Burdock Tea

Ingredients

1 teaspoon of Echinacea powder

1 teaspoon of Burdock root

1-2 cups of hot water

1 teaspoon of honey (optional)

Instructions

Steep the Echinacea powder and the Burdock root in hot water for 7-10 minutes.

Strain, add honey (optional), and drink this aromatic tea!

Remedy 2   Calendula and Licorice Tea

Ingredients

1 teaspoon of Calendula flowers

1 teaspoon of Licorice root

1-2 cups of hot water

1 teaspoon of honey (optional)

Instructions

Steep the Calendula flowers and the Licorice root in hot water for 7-10 minutes.

Strain, add honey (optional), and drink this aromatic tea!

Remedy 3   Marshmallow Root Tea

Ingredients

1 teaspoon of Marshmallow root

1 cup of hot water

1 teaspoon of honey (optional)

Instructions

Steep the Marshmallow root in hot water for 7-10 minutes.

Strain, add honey (optional), and drink this soothing tea!

Remedy 4   Turmeric Root Tea

Ingredients

1 teaspoon of Turmeric root

1 cup of hot water

1 teaspoon of honey (optional)

Instructions

Steep the Turmeric root in hot water for 7-10 minutes.

Strain, add honey (optional), and drink this soothing tea!

Remedy 5   Lavender and Cassia Alata Tea

Ingredients

½ teaspoon of Lavender flowers

½ teaspoon of Cassia Alata seeds

1-2 cups of hot water

1 teaspoon of honey (optional)

Instructions

Steep both herbs together in hot water for 5-10 minutes.

Strain, add honey (optional), and drink this pleasant tea!

Remedy 6   Cassia Alata and Calendula Tea

Ingredients

½ teaspoon of Cassia Alata seeds

½ teaspoon of Calendula flowers

1-2 cups of hot water

1 teaspoon of honey (optional)

Instructions

Steep both herbs together in hot water for 5-10 minutes.

Strain, add honey (optional), and drink this pleasant tea!

Remedy 7   Watermelon Natural Fruit Juice

Ingredients

½ cup of Watermelon (Diced and seeded)

1 teaspoon of Green Tea Powder

2 Tablespoons of honey (optional)

1 cup of water

Instructions

Blend the ingredients

Pour the juice into a glass.

Drink this nourishing juice!

Remedy 8   Grape Natural Fruit Juice

Ingredients

½ cup of Grapes (Stemmed)

1 teaspoon of Calendula Powder

2 Tablespoons of honey (optional)

1 cup of water

Instructions

Blend the ingredients.

Pour the juice into a glass.

Drink this nourishing juice!

Remedy 9   Lavender Herbal Skin Oil

Ingredients

10 drops of Lavender Essential Oil

4 Tablespoons of Cassia Alata infused-Olive Oil

Instructions

Combine the ingredients in an airtight glass dropper bottle.

Shake well for the oils to mix thoroughly.

Use this rejuvenating oil on your skin and the affected area(s)!

Remedy 10 Rosemary Herbal Skin Oil

Ingredients

10 drops of Rosemary Essential Oil

4 Tablespoons of Cassia Alata infused-Calendula Oil

Instructions

Combine the ingredients in an airtight glass dropper bottle.

Shake well for the oils to mix thoroughly.

Use this rejuvenating oil on your skin and the affected area(s)!

Remedy 11 Tea Tree Herbal Skin Oil

Ingredients

10 drops of Tea Tree Essential Oil

4 Tablespoons of Cassia Alata infused-Hemp Seed Oil

Instructions

Combine the ingredients in an airtight glass dropper bottle.

Shake well for the oils to mix thoroughly.

Use this rejuvenating oil on your skin and the affected area(s)!

Remedy 12 Geranium Herbal Skin Oil

Ingredients

10 drops of Geranium Essential Oil

4 Tablespoons of Cassia Alata infused-Rosehip Seed Oil

Instructions

Combine the ingredients in an airtight glass dropper bottle.

Shake well for the oils to mix thoroughly.

Use this rejuvenating oil on your skin and the affected area(s)!

- **Bonus Tips:** manage stress levels well; Avoid direct skin contact with lesions.

ECZEMA

Remedy 1   Cassia Alata and Echinacea Tea

Ingredients

1 teaspoon of Cassia Alata seeds

1 teaspoon of Echinacea root

1-2 cups of hot water

1 teaspoon of honey (optional)

Instructions

Steep the Cassia Alata seeds and the Echinacea root in hot water for 7-10 minutes.

Strain, add honey (optional), and drink this aromatic tea!

Remedy 2   Neem and Burdock Tea

Ingredients

1 teaspoon of Neem powder

1 teaspoon of Burdock root

1-2 cups of hot water

1 teaspoon of honey (optional)

Instructions

Steep the Neem powder and the Burdock root in hot water for 7-10 minutes.

Strain, add honey (optional), and drink this aromatic tea!

Remedy 3   Echinacea Root Tea

Ingredients

1 teaspoon of Echinacea root

1 cup of hot water

1 teaspoon of honey (optional)

Instructions

Steep the Echinacea root in hot water for 7-10 minutes.

Strain, add honey (optional), and drink this soothing tea!

Remedy 4   Horseradish Root Tea

Ingredients

1 teaspoon of Horseradish root

1 cup of hot water

1 teaspoon of honey (optional)

Instructions

Steep the Horseradish root in hot water for 7-10 minutes.

Strain, add honey (optional), and drink this soothing tea!

Remedy 5   Cassia Alata and Neem Tea

Ingredients

½ teaspoon of Cassia Alata seeds

½ teaspoon of Neem powder

1-2 cups of hot water

1 teaspoon of honey (optional)

Instructions

Steep both herbs together in hot water for 5-10 minutes.

Strain, add honey (optional), and drink this pleasant tea!

Remedy 6   Thyme and Ginger Tea

Ingredients

½ teaspoon of Thyme powder

½ teaspoon of Ginger powder

1-2 cups of hot water

1 teaspoon of honey (optional)

Instructions

Steep both herbal powders together in hot water for 5-10 minutes.

Strain, add honey (optional), and drink this pleasant tea!

Remedy 7   Strawberry Natural Fruit Juice

Ingredients

½ cup of Strawberries (Hulled and sliced)

1 teaspoon of Lemon Balm Powder

2 Tablespoons of honey (optional)

1 cup of water

Instructions

Blend the ingredients.

Pour the juice into a glass.

Drink this nourishing juice!

Remedy 8   Kiwi Natural Fruit Juice

Ingredients

½ cup of Kiwi (Peeled and sliced)

1 teaspoon of Echinacea Powder

2 Tablespoons of honey (optional)

1 cup of water

Instructions

Blend the ingredients.

Pour the juice into a glass.

Drink this nourishing juice!

Remedy 9   Chamomile Herbal Skin Oil

Ingredients

10 drops of Chamomile Essential Oil

4 Tablespoons of Cassia Alata infused-Jojoba Oil

Instructions

Combine the ingredients in an airtight glass dropper bottle.

Shake well for the oils to mix thoroughly.

Use this rejuvenating oil on your skin and the affected area(s)!

Remedy 10 Ylang Ylang Herbal Skin Oil

Ingredients

10 drops of Ylang Ylang Essential Oil

4 Tablespoons of Cassia Alata infused-Argan Oil

Instructions

Combine the ingredients in an airtight glass dropper bottle.

Shake well for the oils to mix thoroughly.

Use this rejuvenating oil on your skin and the affected area(s)!

Remedy 11 Frankincense Herbal Skin Oil

Ingredients

10 drops of Frankincense Essential Oil

4 Tablespoons of Cassia Alata infused-Sweet Almond Oil

Instructions

Combine the ingredients in an airtight glass dropper bottle.

Shake well for the oils to mix thoroughly.

Use this rejuvenating oil on your skin and the affected area(s)!

Remedy 12 Eucalyptus Herbal Skin Oil

Ingredients

10 drops of Eucalyptus Essential Oil

4 Tablespoons of Cassia Alata infused-Grapeseed Oil

Instructions

Combine the ingredients in an airtight glass dropper bottle.

Shake well for the oils to mix thoroughly.

Use this rejuvenating oil on your skin and the affected area(s)!

- o **Bonus Tips:** keep skin properly moisturized; avoid allergens.

ASTHMA

Remedy 1   Fennel Seed and Ginger Tea

Ingredients

1 teaspoon of Fennel seed powder

1 teaspoon of Ginger root

1-2 cups of hot water

1 teaspoon of honey (optional)

Instructions

Steep the seed Fennel powder and the Ginger root in hot water for 10-15 minutes.

Strain, add honey (optional), and drink this wonderful tea!

Remedy 2   Flaxseed and Licorice Tea

Ingredients

1 teaspoon of Flaxseed powder

1 teaspoon of Licorice root

1-2 cups of hot water

1 teaspoon of honey (optional)

Instructions

Steep the Flaxseed powder and the Licorice root in hot water for 10-15 minutes.

Strain, add honey (optional), and drink this wonderful tea!

Remedy 3   Lavender Flowers Tea

Ingredients

1 Tablespoon of Lavender flowers

1 cup of hot water

1 teaspoon of honey (optional)

Instructions

Steep the Lavender flowers in hot water for 10-15 minutes.

Strain, add honey (optional), and drink this floral tea!

Remedy 4   Chamomile Flowers Tea

Ingredients

1 Tablespoon of Chamomile flowers

1 cup of hot water

1 teaspoon of honey (optional)

Instructions

Steep the Chamomile flowers in hot water for 10-15 minutes.

Strain, add honey (optional), and drink this floral tea!

Remedy 5   Peppermint Leaf Tea

Ingredients

1 Tablespoon of Peppermint leaves

1 cup of hot water

1 teaspoon of honey (optional)

Instructions

Steep the Peppermint leaves in hot water for 10-15 minutes.

Strain, add honey (optional), and drink this aromatic tea!

Remedy 6   Oregano Leaf Tea

Ingredients

1 Tablespoon of Oregano leaves

1 cup of hot water

1 teaspoon of honey (optional)

Instructions

Steep the Oregano leaves in hot water for 10-15 minutes.

Strain, add honey (optional), and drink this aromatic tea!

Remedy 7   Red Root Tea

Ingredients

1 teaspoon of Red root

1 cup of hot water

1 teaspoon of honey (optional)

Instructions

Steep the Red root in hot water for 7-10 minutes.

Strain, add honey (optional), and drink this soothing tea!

Remedy 8   Marshmallow Root Tea

Ingredients

1 teaspoon of Marshmallow root

1 cup of hot water

1 teaspoon of honey (optional)

Instructions

Steep the Marshmallow root in hot water for 7-10 minutes.

Strain, add honey (optional), and drink this soothing tea!

Remedy 9   Berry-Blend Natural Fruit Juice

Ingredients

½ cup of Blueberries

½ cup of Raspberries

1 teaspoon of Mullein Powder

2 Tablespoons of honey (optional)

1-2 cups of water

Instructions

Blend the ingredients.

Pour the juice into a glass.

Drink this sparkling juice!

Remedy 10 Berry-Mix Natural Fruit Juice

Ingredients

½ cup of Strawberries (Hulled and sliced)

½ cup of Blackberries

1 teaspoon of Ginseng Powder

2 Tablespoons of honey (optional)

1-2 cups of water

Instructions

Blend the ingredients.

Pour the juice into a glass.

Drink this sparkling juice!

Remedy 11 Tea Tree Aromatherapy

Ingredients

7 drops of Tea Tree Essential Oil

5 drops of Orange Essential Oil

Distilled water (for Diffuser)

Instructions

Combine the Essential Oils in a glass dropper bottle, and mix well.

Fill the diffuser with the distilled water.

Add a few drops of this Essential Oil blend to the distilled water.

Turn on the diffuser.

Remain in this relaxing aroma for at least 20 minutes.

Remedy 12 Lavender Aromatherapy

Ingredients

8 drops of Lavender Essential Oil

8 drops of Lemongrass Essential Oil

Distilled water (for Diffuser)

Instructions

Combine the Essential Oils in a glass dropper bottle, and mix well.

Fill the diffuser with the distilled water.

Add a few drops of this Essential Oil blend to the distilled water.

Turn on the diffuser.

Remain in this relaxing aroma for at least 20 minutes.

- **Bonus Tips:** keep your environment clean; avoid exposure to dust and other allergens.

THE COMMON FLU

Remedy 1 Sunflower Seed and Ginger Tea

Ingredients

1 teaspoon of Sunflower seed powder

1 teaspoon of Ginger root

1-2 cups of hot water

1 teaspoon of honey (optional)

Instructions

Steep the Sunflower seed powder and the Ginger root in hot water for 10-15 minutes.

Strain, add honey (optional), and drink this wonderful tea!

Remedy 2   Sesame Seed and Echinacea Tea

Ingredients

1 teaspoon of Sesame seed powder

1 teaspoon of Echinacea root

1-2 cups of hot water

1 teaspoon of honey (optional)

Instructions

Steep the Sesame seed powder and the Echinacea root in hot water for 10-15 minutes.

Strain, add honey (optional), and drink this wonderful tea!

Remedy 3   Yarrow Flowers Tea

Ingredients

1 Tablespoon of Yarrow flowers

1 cup of hot water

1 teaspoon of honey (optional)

Instructions

Steep the Yarrow flowers in hot water for 10-15 minutes.

Strain, add honey (optional), and drink this floral tea!

Remedy 4   Elderflowers Tea

Ingredients

1 Tablespoon of Elderflowers

1 cup of hot water

1 teaspoon of honey (optional)

Instructions

Steep the Elderflowers in hot water for 10-15 minutes.

Strain, add honey (optional), and drink this floral tea!

Remedy 5   Peppermint Leaf Tea

Ingredients

1 Tablespoon of Peppermint leaves

1 cup of hot water

1 teaspoon of honey (optional)

Instructions

Steep the Peppermint leaves in hot water for 10-15 minutes.

Strain, add honey (optional), and drink this aromatic tea!

Remedy 6   Thyme Leaf Tea

Ingredients

1 Tablespoon of Thyme leaves

1 cup of hot water

1 teaspoon of honey (optional)

Instructions

Steep the Thyme leaves in hot water for 10-15 minutes.

Strain, add honey (optional), and drink this aromatic tea!

Remedy 7 Osha Root Tea

Ingredients

1 teaspoon of Osha root

1 cup of hot water

1 teaspoon of honey (optional)

Instructions

Steep the Osha root in hot water for 7-10 minutes.

Strain, add honey (optional), and drink this soothing tea!

Remedy 8   Astralagus Root Tea

Ingredients

1 teaspoon of Astralagus root

1 cup of hot water

1 teaspoon of honey (optional)

Instructions

Steep the Astralagus root in hot water for 7-10 minutes.

Strain, add honey (optional), and drink this soothing tea!

Remedy 9   Natural Fruit Juice Mix

Ingredients

½ cup of Pomegranate (Seeds extracted)

½ cup of Kiwi (Peeled and sliced)

1 teaspoon of Nettle Powder

2 Tablespoons of honey (optional)

1-2 cups of water

Instructions

Blend the ingredients.

Pour the juice into a glass.

Drink this sparkling juice!

Remedy 10 Natural Fruit Juice Blend

Ingredients

½ cup of Cantaloupe (Peeled, seeded, and diced)

½ cup of Strawberry (Hulled and sliced)

1 teaspoon of Ginger Powder

2 Tablespoons of honey (optional)

1-2 cups of water

Instructions

Blend the ingredients.

Pour the juice into a glass.

Drink this sparkling juice!

Remedy 11 Peppermint Aromatherapy

Ingredients

5 drops of Peppermint Essential Oil

7 drops of Lavender Essential Oil

Distilled water (for Diffuser)

Instructions

Combine the Essential Oils in a glass dropper bottle, and mix well.

Fill the diffuser with the distilled water.

Add a few drops of this Essential Oil blend to the distilled water.

Turn on the diffuser.

Remain in this relaxing aroma for at least 20 minutes.

Remedy 12 Eucalyptus Aromatherapy

Ingredients

8 drops of Eucalyptus Essential Oil

8 drops of Lemongrass Essential Oil

Distilled water (for Diffuser)

Instructions

Combine the Essential Oils in a glass dropper bottle, and mix well.

Fill the diffuser with the distilled water.

Add a few drops of this Essential Oil blend to the distilled water.

Turn on the diffuser.

Remain in this relaxing aroma for at least 20 minutes.

- **Bonus Tips:** practice proper hygiene; consume herbal suggestions that prevent and eradicate the Flu.

GLAUCOMA

Remedy 1 Bilberry and Eyebright Tea

Ingredients

½ teaspoon of Bilberry powder

½ teaspoon of Eyebright powder

1-2 cups of hot water

1 teaspoon of honey (optional)

Instructions

Steep both herbal powders together in hot water for 5-10 minutes.

Strain, add honey (optional), and drink this pleasant tea!

Remedy 2   Calendula and Fennel Tea

Ingredients

½ teaspoon of Calendula flowers

½ teaspoon of Fennel seeds

1-2 cups of hot water

1 teaspoon of honey (optional)

Instructions

Steep both herbs together in hot water for 7-10 minutes.

Strain, add honey (optional), and drink this pleasant tea!

Remedy 3   Ginkgo Biloba and Rosemary Tea

Ingredients

½ teaspoon of Ginkgo Biloba powder

½ teaspoon of Rosemary powder

1-2 cups of hot water

1 teaspoon of honey (optional)

Instructions

Steep both herbal powders together in hot water for 5-10 minutes.

Strain, add honey (optional), and drink this pleasant tea!

Remedy 4   Eyebright and Elderberry Tea

Ingredients

½ teaspoon of Eyebright powder

½ teaspoon of Elderberry powder

1-2 cups of hot water

1 teaspoon of honey (optional)

Instructions

Steep both herbal powders together in hot water for 5-10 minutes.

Strain, add honey (optional), and drink this pleasant tea!

Remedy 5   Green Tea and Passionflower Tea

Ingredients

½ teaspoon of Green Tea powder

½ teaspoon of Passionflower powder

1-2 cups of hot water

1 teaspoon of honey (optional)

Instructions

Steep both herbal powders together in hot water for 5-10 minutes.

Strain, add honey (optional), and drink this pleasant tea!

Remedy 6   Ginkgo Biloba and Eyebright Tea

Ingredients

½ teaspoon of Ginkgo Biloba powder

½ teaspoon of Eyebright powder

1-2 cups of hot water

1 teaspoon of honey (optional)

Instructions

Steep both herbal powders together in hot water for 5-10 minutes.

Strain, add honey (optional), and drink this pleasant tea!

Remedy 7   Ginkgo Biloba Eye drop

Ingredients

1 cup of hot water and 1 teaspoon of Ginkgo Biloba leaves.

Instructions

Place the Ginkgo Biloba leaves into a teapot and pour the hot water over it.

Allow to steep and cool for 25-30 minutes.

Strain well to remove herb particles.

Place this eye wash into a clean sterile glass dropper bottle.

Tilt your head backward.

Insert 1-2 drops of this eye wash into each eye at least twice daily.

Ensure that the eyewash is clean and fresh before every use.

Remedy 8   Fennel Eye drop

Ingredients

1 cup of hot water and 1 teaspoon of Fennel seeds.

Instructions

Place the Fennel seeds into a teapot and pour the hot water over it.

Allow to steep and cool for 25-30 minutes.

Strain well to remove herb particles.

Place this eye wash into a clean sterile glass dropper bottle.

Tilt your head backward.

Insert 1-2 drops of this eye wash into each eye at least twice daily.

Ensure that the eyewash is clean and fresh before every use.

Remedy 9   Yarrow Eye drop

Ingredients

1 cup of hot water and 1 teaspoon of Yarrow leaves.

Instructions

Place the Yarrow leaves into a teapot and pour the hot water over it.

Allow to steep and cool for 25-30 minutes.

Strain well to remove herb particles.

Place this eye wash into a clean sterile glass dropper bottle.

Tilt your head backward.

Insert 1-2 drops of this eye wash into each eye at least twice daily.

Ensure that the eyewash is clean and fresh before every use.

Remedy 10 Goldenrod Eye Drop

Ingredients

1 cup of hot water and 1 teaspoon of Goldenrod leaves.

Instructions

Place the Goldenrod leaves into a teapot and pour the hot water over it.

Allow to steep and cool for 25-30 minutes.

Strain well to remove herb particles.

Place this eye wash into a clean sterile glass dropper bottle.

Tilt your head backward.

Insert 1-2 drops of this eye wash into each eye at least twice daily.

Ensure that the eyewash is clean and fresh before every use.

Remedy 11 Zesty Natural Fruit Juice

Ingredients

½ cup of Strawberries (Hulled and sliced)

½ cup of Grapes (Stemmed)

1 teaspoon of Ginkgo Biloba Powder

2 Tablespoons of honey (optional)

1-2 cups of water

Instructions

Blend the ingredients.

Pour the juice into a glass.

Drink this sparkling juice!

Remedy 12 Natural Fruit Juice Delight

Ingredients

½ cup of Orange (Peeled and segmented)

½ cup of Cranberries

1 teaspoon of Eyebright Powder

2 Tablespoons of honey (optional)

1-2 cups of water

Instructions

Blend the ingredients.

Pour the juice into a glass.

Drink this sparkling juice!

- **Bonus Tips:** continue with proper eye care diet and practices; continue with proper eye care exercises.

CATARACT

Remedy 1   Milk Thistle and Eyebright Tea

Ingredients

½ teaspoon of Milk Thistle powder

½ teaspoon of Eyebright powder

1-2 cups of hot water

1 teaspoon of honey (optional)

Instructions

Steep both herbal powders together in hot water for 5-10 minutes.

Strain, add honey (optional), and drink this pleasant tea!

Remedy 2   Schisandra and Astragalus Tea

Ingredients

½ teaspoon of Schisandra powder

½ teaspoon of Astragalus powder

1-2 cups of hot water

1 teaspoon of honey (optional)

Instructions

Steep both herbal powders together in hot water for 5-10 minutes.

Strain, add honey (optional), and drink this pleasant tea!

Remedy 3   Alfalfa and Green Tea

Ingredients

½ teaspoon of Alfalfa powder

½ teaspoon of Green Tea powder

1-2 cups of hot water

1 teaspoon of honey (optional)

Instructions

Steep both herbal powders together in hot water for 5-10 minutes.

Strain, add honey (optional), and drink this pleasant tea!

Remedy 4   Dill and Goldenseal Tea

Ingredients

½ teaspoon of Dill powder

½ teaspoon of Goldenseal powder

1-2 cups of hot water

1 teaspoon of honey (optional)

Instructions

Steep both herbal powders together in hot water for 5-10 minutes.

Strain, add honey (optional), and drink this pleasant tea!

Remedy 5   Eyebright and Butcher's Broom Tea

Ingredients

½ teaspoon of Eyebright powder

½ teaspoon of Butcher's Broom powder

1-2 cups of hot water

1 teaspoon of honey (optional)

Instructions

Steep both herbal powders together in hot water for 5-10 minutes.

Strain, add honey (optional), and drink this pleasant tea!

Remedy 6 Hawthorn and Juniper Berry Tea

Ingredients

½ teaspoon of Hawthorn powder

½ teaspoon of Juniper Berry powder

1-2 cups of hot water

1 teaspoon of honey (optional)

Instructions

Steep both herbal powders together in hot water for 5-10 minutes.

Strain, add honey (optional), and drink this pleasant tea!

Remedy 7 Eyebright Eye drop

Ingredients

1 cup of hot water and 1 teaspoon of Eyebright leaves.

Instructions

Place the Eyebright leaves into a teapot and pour the hot water over it.

Allow to steep and cool for 25-30 minutes.

Strain well to remove herb particles.

Place this eye wash into a clean sterile glass dropper bottle.

Tilt your head backward.

Insert 1-2 drops of this eye wash into each eye at least twice daily.

Ensure that the eyewash is clean and fresh before every use.

Remedy 8   Fennel Eye drop

Ingredients

1 cup of hot water and 1 teaspoon of Fennel seeds.

Instructions

Place the Fennel seeds into a teapot and pour the hot water over it.

Allow to steep and cool for 25-30 minutes.

Strain well to remove herb particles.

Place this eye wash into a clean sterile glass dropper bottle.

Tilt your head backward.

Insert 1-2 drops of this eye wash into each eye at least twice daily.

Ensure that the eyewash is clean and fresh before every use.

Remedy 9   Milk Thistle Eye drop

Ingredients

1 cup of hot water and 1 teaspoon of Milk Thistle leaves.

Instructions

Place the Milk Thistle leaves into a teapot and pour the hot water over it.

Allow to steep and cool for 25-30 minutes.

Strain well to remove herb particles.

Place this eye wash into a clean sterile glass dropper bottle.

Tilt your head backward.

Insert 1-2 drops of this eye wash into each eye at least twice daily.

Ensure that the eyewash is clean and fresh before every use.

Remedy 10 Chamomile Eye drop

Ingredients

1 cup of hot water and 1 teaspoon of Chamomile flowers.

Instructions

Place the Chamomile flowers into a teapot and pour the hot water over it.

Allow to steep and cool for 25-30 minutes.

Strain well to remove herb particles.

Place this eye wash into a clean sterile glass dropper bottle.

Tilt your head backward.

Insert 1-2 drops of this eye wash into each eye at least twice daily.

Ensure that the eyewash is clean and fresh before every use.

Remedy 11 Natural Fruit Juice World

Ingredients

½ cup of Apricots (Peeled, pitted, and sliced)

½ cup of Apples (Cored and sliced)

1 teaspoon of Green Tea Powder

2 Tablespoons of honey (optional)

1-2 cups of water

Instructions

Blend the ingredients.

Pour the juice into a glass.

Drink this sparkling juice!

Remedy 12 Tropical Natural Fruit Juice

Ingredients

½ cup of Banana (Peeled and sliced)

½ cup of Papaya (Peeled, seeded, and diced)

1 teaspoon of Hibiscus Powder

2 Tablespoons of honey (optional)

1-2 cups of water

Instructions

Blend the ingredients.

Pour the juice into a glass.

Drink this sparkling juice!

- o **Bonus Tips:** continue with proper eye care diet and practices; continue with proper eye care exercises.

EAR ACHE

Remedy 1   Olive Oil Ear Drop

Ingredients

2-3 drops of Thyme Essential Oil

1-2 drops of Rosemary Essential Oil

4 teaspoons of Olive Oil

Instructions

Place the ingredients into a clean sterile glass dropper bottle.

Ensure the bottle is sealed tight, and shake well to mix the ingredients thoroughly.

Tilt your head so the affected ear is facing upwards.

Insert 2-3 drops of this oil mixture into the affected ear twice daily.

Store this oil in a cool dark place.

Remedy 2   Sunflower Seed Oil Ear Drop

Ingredients

2-3 drops of Tea Tree Essential Oil

1-2 drops of Lavender Essential Oil

4 teaspoons of Sunflower Seed Oil

Instructions

Place the ingredients into a clean sterile glass dropper bottle.

Ensure the bottle is sealed tight, and shake well to mix the ingredients thoroughly.

Tilt your head so the affected ear is facing upwards.

Insert 2-3 drops of this oil mixture into the affected ear twice daily.

Store this oil in a cool dark place.

Remedy 3   Coconut Oil Ear Drop

Ingredients

2-3 drops of Lavender Essential Oil

1-2 drops of Eucalyptus Essential Oil

4 teaspoons of Coconut Oil

Instructions

Place the ingredients into a clean sterile glass dropper bottle.

Ensure the bottle is sealed tight, and shake well to mix the ingredients thoroughly.

Tilt your head so the affected ear is facing upwards.

Insert 2-3 drops of this oil mixture into the affected ear twice daily.

Store this oil in a cool dark place.

Remedy 4   Grapeseed Oil Ear Drop

Ingredients

2-3 drops of Rosemary Essential Oil

1-2 drops of Oregano Essential Oil

4 teaspoons of Grapeseed Oil

Instructions

Place the ingredients into a clean sterile glass dropper bottle.

Ensure the bottle is sealed tight, and shake well to mix the ingredients thoroughly.

Tilt your head so the affected ear is facing upwards.

Insert 2-3 drops of this oil mixture into the affected ear twice daily.

Store this oil in a cool dark place.

Remedy 5   Jojoba Ear Massage Oil

Ingredients

2-3 drops of Lavender Essential Oil

1-2 drops of Wintergreen Essential Oil

4 teaspoons of Jojoba Oil

Instructions

Place the ingredients into a clean sterile glass dropper bottle.

Ensure the bottle is sealed tight, and shake well to mix the ingredients thoroughly.

Gently massage the affected ear(s) with this oil.

Store this oil in a cool dark place.

Remedy 6   Argan Ear Massage Oil

Ingredients

2-3 drops of Lemongrass Essential Oil

1-2 drops of Lemon Essential Oil

4 teaspoons of Argan Oil

Instructions

Place the ingredients into a clean sterile glass dropper bottle.

Ensure the bottle is sealed tight, and shake well to mix the ingredients thoroughly.

Gently massage the affected ear(s) with this oil.

Store this oil in a cool dark place.

Remedy 7   Rosemary Ear Massage Oil

Ingredients

2-3 drops of Sweet Orange Essential Oil

1-2 drops of Tea Tree Essential Oil

4 teaspoons of Rosemary infused-Olive Oil

Instructions

Place the ingredients into a clean sterile glass dropper bottle.

Ensure the bottle is sealed tight, and shake well to mix the ingredients thoroughly.

Gently massage the affected ear(s) with this oil.

Store this oil in a cool dark place.

Remedy 8   Hemp Seed Ear Massage Oil

Ingredients

2-3 drops of Basil Essential Oil

1-2 drops of Tea Tree Essential Oil

4 teaspoons of Hemp Seed Oil

Instructions

Place the ingredients into a clean sterile glass dropper bottle.

Ensure the bottle is sealed tight, and shake well to mix the ingredients thoroughly.

Gently massage the affected ear(s) with this oil.

Store this oil in a cool dark place.

Remedy 9   Garlic and Ginger Root Tea

Ingredients

1 teaspoon of Garlic powder

1 teaspoon of Ginger root

1-2 cups of hot water

1 teaspoon of honey (optional)

Instructions

Steep the Garlic powder and the Ginger root in hot water for 7-10 minutes.

Strain, add honey (optional), and drink this aromatic tea!

Remedy 10 Sage and Cat's Claw Root Tea

Ingredients

1 teaspoon of Sage powder

1 teaspoon of Cat's Claw root

1-2 cups of hot water

1 teaspoon of honey (optional)

Instructions

Steep the Sage powder and the Cat's Claw root in hot water for 7-10 minutes.

Strain, add honey (optional), and drink this aromatic tea!

Remedy 11 Grapefruit Natural Fruit Juice

Ingredients

½ cup of Grapefruit (Peeled and segmented)

1 teaspoon of Horsetail Powder

2 Tablespoons of honey (optional)

1 cup of water

Instructions

Blend the ingredients.

Pour the juice into a glass.

Drink this nourishing juice!

Remedy 12 Plum Natural Fruit Juice

Ingredients

½ cup of Plum (Pitted and sliced)

1 teaspoon of Lemon Verbena Powder

2 Tablespoons of honey (optional)

1 cup of water

Instructions

Blend the ingredients.

Pour the juice into a glass.

Drink this nourishing juice!

- **Bonus Tips:** a warm compress applied to the outer ear helps; avoid inserting objects into the ear canal.

EAR INFECTION

Remedy 1 **Tea Tree Oil Ear Drop**

Ingredients

2-3 drops of Tea Tree Essential Oil

1-2 drops of Peppermint Essential Oil

4 teaspoons of Coconut Oil

Instructions

Place the ingredients into a clean sterile glass dropper bottle.

Ensure the bottle is sealed tight, and shake well to mix the ingredients thoroughly.

Tilt your head so the affected ear is facing upwards.

Insert 2-3 drops of this oil mixture into the affected ear twice daily.

Store this oil in a cool dark place.

Remedy 2   Lavender Oil Ear Drop

Ingredients

2-3 drops of Lavender Essential Oil

1-2 drops of Rosemary Essential Oil

4 teaspoons of Jojoba Oil

Instructions

Place the ingredients into a clean sterile glass dropper bottle.

Ensure the bottle is sealed tight, and shake well to mix the ingredients thoroughly.

Tilt your head so the affected ear is facing upwards.

Insert 2-3 drops of this oil mixture into the affected ear twice daily.

Store this oil in a cool dark place.

Remedy 3   Thyme Oil Ear Drop

Ingredients

2-3 drops of Thyme Essential Oil

1-2 drops of Orange Essential Oil

4 teaspoons of Olive Oil

Instructions

Place the ingredients into a clean sterile glass dropper bottle.

Ensure the bottle is sealed tight, and shake well to mix the ingredients thoroughly.

Tilt your head so the affected ear is facing upwards.

Insert 2-3 drops of this oil mixture into the affected ear twice daily.

Store this oil in a cool dark place.

Remedy 4   Eucalyptus Oil Ear Drop

Ingredients

2-3 drops of Eucalyptus Essential Oil

1-2 drops of Peppermint Essential Oil

4 teaspoons of Argan Oil

Instructions

Place the ingredients into a clean sterile glass dropper bottle.

Ensure the bottle is sealed tight, and shake well to mix the ingredients thoroughly.

Tilt your head so the affected ear is facing upwards.

Insert 2-3 drops of this oil mixture into the affected ear twice daily.

Store this oil in a cool dark place.

Remedy 5   Basil Ear Massage Oil

Ingredients

2-3 drops of Chamomile Essential Oil

1-2 drops of Basil Essential Oil

4 teaspoons of Sunflower Seed Oil

Instructions

Place the ingredients into a clean sterile glass dropper bottle.

Ensure the bottle is sealed tight, and shake well to mix the ingredients thoroughly.

Tilt your head so the affected ear is facing upwards.

Insert 2-3 drops of this oil mixture into the affected ear twice daily.

Store this oil in a cool dark place.

Remedy 6   Clove Ear Massage Oil

Ingredients

2-3 drops of Oregano Essential Oil

1-2 drops of Clove Essential Oil

4 teaspoons of Grapeseed Oil

Instructions

Place the ingredients into a clean sterile glass dropper bottle.

Ensure the bottle is sealed tight, and shake well to mix the ingredients thoroughly.

Tilt your head so the affected ear is facing upwards.

Insert 2-3 drops of this oil mixture into the affected ear twice daily.

Store this oil in a cool dark place.

Remedy 7   Frankincense Ear Massage Oil

Ingredients

2-3 drops of Lemon Essential Oil

1-2 drops of Frankincense Essential Oil

4 teaspoons of Rosemary infused-Olive Oil

Instructions

Place the ingredients into a clean sterile glass dropper bottle.

Ensure the bottle is sealed tight, and shake well to mix the ingredients thoroughly.

Tilt your head so the affected ear is facing upwards.

Insert 2-3 drops of this oil mixture into the affected ear twice daily.

Store this oil in a cool dark place.

Remedy 8   Lemongrass Ear Massage Oil

Ingredients

2-3 drops of Myrrh Essential Oil

1-2 drops of Lemongrass Essential Oil

4 teaspoons of Argan Oil

Instructions

Place the ingredients into a clean sterile glass dropper bottle.

Ensure the bottle is sealed tight, and shake well to mix the ingredients thoroughly.

Tilt your head so the affected ear is facing upwards.

Insert 2-3 drops of this oil mixture into the affected ear twice daily.

Store this oil in a cool dark place.

Remedy 9   Yellow Dock and Echinacea Root Tea

Ingredients

1 teaspoon of Yellow Dock powder

1 teaspoon of Echinacea root

1-2 cups of hot water

1 teaspoon of honey (optional)

Instructions

Steep the Yellow Dock powder and the Echinacea root in hot water for 7-10 minutes.

Strain, add honey (optional), and drink this aromatic tea!

Remedy 10 Black Walnut and Echinacea Root Tea

Ingredients

1 teaspoon of Black Walnut powder

1 teaspoon of Echinacea root

1-2 cups of hot water

1 teaspoon of honey (optional)

Instructions

Steep the Black Walnut powder and the Echinacea root in hot water for 7-10 minutes.

Strain, add honey (optional), and drink this aromatic tea!

Remedy 11 Watermelon Natural Fruit Juice

Ingredients

½ cup of Watermelon (Diced and seeded)

1 teaspoon of Peppermint Powder

2 Tablespoons of honey (optional)

1 cup of water

Instructions

Blend the ingredients.

Pour the juice into a glass.

Drink this nourishing juice!

Remedy 12 Pomegranate Natural Fruit Juice

Ingredients

½ cup of Pomegranate (Seeds extracted)

1 teaspoon of Lavender Powder

2 Tablespoons of honey (optional)

1 cup of water

Instructions

Blend the ingredients.

Pour the juice into a glass.

Drink this nourishing juice!

- **Bonus Tips:** keep ears clean at all times; avoid ear irritants.

DEPRESSION

Remedy 1   Ginkgo Biloba and Ginseng Root Tea

Ingredients

1 teaspoon of Ginkgo Biloba powder

1 teaspoon of Ginseng root

1-2 cups of hot water

1 teaspoon of honey (optional)

Instructions

Steep the Ginkgo Biloba powder and the Ginseng root in hot water for 7-10 minutes.

Strain, add honey (optional), and drink this aromatic tea!

Remedy 2   Ginger Root Tea

Ingredients

1 teaspoon of Ginger root

1 cup of hot water

1 teaspoon of honey (optional)

Instructions:

Steep the Ginger root in hot water for 7-10 minutes.

Strain, add honey (optional), and drink this soothing tea!

Remedy 3   Ginger Root and Turmeric Root Tea

Ingredients

1 teaspoon of Ginger root

1 teaspoon of Turmeric root

1-2 cups of hot water

1 teaspoon of honey (optional)

Instructions

Steep both herbal roots in hot water for 7-10 minutes.

Strain, add honey (optional), and drink this delightful tea!

Remedy 4   Flaxseed and Licorice Root Tea

Ingredients

1 teaspoon of Flaxseed powder

1 teaspoon of Licorice root

1-2 cups of hot water

1 teaspoon of honey (optional)

Instructions

Steep the Flaxseed powder and the Licorice root in hot water for 10-15 minutes.

Strain, add honey (optional), and drink this wonderful tea!

Remedy 5   Rosemary and Licorice Tea

Ingredients

½ teaspoon of Rosemary powder

½ teaspoon of Licorice powder

1-2 cups of hot water

1 teaspoon of honey (optional)

Instructions

Steep both herbal powders together in hot water for 5-10 minutes.

Strain, add honey (optional), and drink this pleasant tea!

Remedy 6   Passionflower Tea

Ingredients

1 Tablespoon of Passionflower

1 cup of hot water

1 teaspoon of honey (optional)

Instructions

Steep the Passionflower in hot water for 10-15 minutes.

Strain, add honey (optional), and drink this floral tea!

Remedy 7   Cantaloupe Natural Fruit Juice

Ingredients

½ cup of Cantaloupe (Peeled, seeded, and diced)

1 teaspoon of Maca Powder

2 Tablespoons of honey (optional)

1 cup of water

Instructions

Blend the ingredients.

Pour the juice into a glass.

Drink this nourishing juice!

Remedy 8   Natural Fruit Juice Twist

Ingredients

½ cup of Mango (Peeled and diced)

½ cup of Blueberries

1 teaspoon of Ginkgo Biloba Powder

2 Tablespoons of honey (optional)

1-2 cups of water

Instructions

Blend the ingredients.

Pour the juice into a glass.

Drink this sparkling juice!

Remedy 9   Cherry Herbal Smoothie

Ingredients

1 teaspoon of powdered Ashwagandha

1-2 Tablespoons of Honey (optional)

1 cup of Cherries (Pitted)

1-2 cups of Almond Milk

Instruction

Combine the ingredients in a blender.

Blend all the ingredients to your desired smooth consistency.

Pour the smoothie into a glass.

Enjoy this delicious smoothie!

Remedy 10 Papaya Herbal Smoothie

Ingredients

1 teaspoon of powdered Kava Kava

1 teaspoon of powdered St. John's Wort

1-2 Tablespoons of Honey (optional)

1 cup of Papaya (Peeled, seeded, and diced)

1-2 cups of Oat Milk

Instructions

Combine the powdered herbs in an airtight container.

Shake well until the powdered herbs are thoroughly mixed.

Combine the ingredients in a blender, along with 1 teaspoon of this herbal powder mixture.

Blend all the ingredients to your desired smooth consistency.

Pour the smoothie into a glass.

Enjoy this delicious smoothie!

Remedy 11 Peppermint Aromatherapy

Ingredients

9 drops of Peppermint Essential Oil

6 drops of Lavender Essential Oil

Distilled water (for Diffuser)

Instructions

Combine the Essential Oils in a glass dropper bottle, and mix well.

Fill the diffuser with the distilled water.

Add a few drops of this Essential Oil blend to the distilled water.

Turn on the diffuser.

Remain in this relaxing aroma for at least 20 minutes.

Remedy 12 Frankincense Aromatherapy

Ingredients

7 drops of Frankincense Essential Oil

8 drops of Ginger Essential Oil

Distilled water (for Diffuser)

Instructions

Combine the Essential Oils in a glass dropper bottle, and mix well.

Fill the diffuser with the distilled water.

Add a few drops of this Essential Oil blend to the distilled water.

Turn on the diffuser.

Remain in this relaxing aroma for at least 20 minutes.

- **Bonus Tips:** be consistent with proper healthcare treatment; be positive.

MIGRAINE

Remedy 1   Ashwagandha and Echinacea Root Tea

Ingredients

1 teaspoon of Ashwagandha powder

1 teaspoon of Echinacea root

1-2 cups of hot water

1 teaspoon of honey (optional)

Instructions

Steep the Ashwagandha powder and the Echinacea root in hot water for 7-10 minutes.

Strain, add honey (optional), and drink this aromatic tea!

Remedy 2 Licorice Root Tea

Ingredients

1 teaspoon of Licorice root

1 cup of hot water

1 teaspoon of honey (optional)

Instructions:

Steep the Licorice root in hot water for 7-10 minutes.

Strain, add honey (optional), and drink this soothing tea!

Remedy 3 Valerian Root and Dandelion Root Tea

Ingredients

1 teaspoon of Valerian root

1 teaspoon of Dandelion root

1-2 cups of hot water

1 teaspoon of honey (optional)

Instructions

Steep both herbal roots in hot water for 7-10 minutes.

Strain, add honey (optional), and drink this delightful tea!

Remedy 4   Chia Seed and Astragalus Root Tea

Ingredients

1 teaspoon of Chia seed powder

1 teaspoon of Astragalus root

1-2 cups of hot water

1 teaspoon of honey (optional)

Instructions

Steep the Chia seed powder and the Astragalus root in hot water for 10-15 minutes.

Strain, add honey (optional), and drink this wonderful tea!

Remedy 5   Gotu Kola and Lemon Balm Tea

Ingredients

½ teaspoon of Gotu Kola powder

½ teaspoon of Lemon Balm powder

1-2 cups of hot water

1 teaspoon of honey (optional)

Instructions

Steep both herbal powders together in hot water for 5-10 minutes.

Strain, add honey (optional), and drink this pleasant tea!

Remedy 6   Chamomile Flowers Tea

Ingredients

1 Tablespoon of Chamomile flowers

1 cup of hot water

1 teaspoon of honey (optional)

Instructions

Steep the Chamomile flowers in hot water for 10-15 minutes.

Strain, add honey (optional), and drink this floral tea!

Remedy 7   Strawberry Natural Fruit Juice

Ingredients

½ cup of Strawberry (Hulled and sliced)

1 teaspoon of Ashwagandha Powder

2 Tablespoons of honey (optional)

1 cup of water

Instructions

Blend the ingredients.

Pour the juice into a glass.

Drink this nourishing juice!

Remedy 8   Flavored Natural Fruit Juice

Ingredients

½ cup of Apple (Cored and sliced)

½ cup of Grapes (Stemmed)

1 teaspoon of Peppermint Powder

2 Tablespoons of honey (optional)

1-2 cups of water

Instructions

Blend the ingredients.

Pour the juice into a glass.

Drink this sparkling juice!

Remedy 9   Pineapple Herbal Smoothie

Ingredients

1 teaspoon of powdered Rhodiola Rosea

1-2 Tablespoons of Honey (optional)

1 cup of Pineapple (Peeled, cored, and diced)

1-2 cups of Almond Milk

Instruction

Combine the ingredients in a blender.

Blend all the ingredients to your desired smooth consistency.

Pour the smoothie into a glass.

Enjoy this delicious smoothie!

Remedy 10 Banana Herbal Smoothie

Ingredients

1 teaspoon of powdered Skullcap

1 teaspoon of powdered St. John's Wort

1-2 Tablespoons of Honey (optional)

1 cup of Banana (Peeled and sliced)

1-2 cups of Oat Milk

Instructions

Combine the powdered herbs in an airtight container.

Shake well until the powdered herbs are thoroughly mixed.

Combine the ingredients in a blender, along with 1 teaspoon of this herbal powder mixture.

Blend all the ingredients to your desired smooth consistency.

Pour the smoothie into a glass.

Enjoy this delicious smoothie!

Remedy 11 Bergamot Aromatherapy

Ingredients

9 drops of Bergamot Essential Oil

6 drops of Basil Essential Oil

Distilled water (for Diffuser)

Instructions

Combine the Essential Oils in a glass dropper bottle, and mix well.

Fill the diffuser with the distilled water.

Add a few drops of this Essential Oil blend to the distilled water.

Turn on the diffuser.

Remain in this relaxing aroma for at least 20 minutes.

Remedy 12 Vetiver Aromatherapy

Ingredients

7 drops of Vetiver Essential Oil

8 drops of Patchouli Essential Oil

Distilled water (for Diffuser)

Instructions

Combine the Essential Oils in a glass dropper bottle, and mix well.

Fill the diffuser with the distilled water.

Add a few drops of this Essential Oil blend to the distilled water.

Turn on the diffuser.

Remain in this relaxing aroma for at least 20 minutes.

- **Bonus Tips:** note and avoid triggers; get adequate sleep and relaxation; drink enough water.

GINGIVITIS

Remedy 1   Spearmint Herbal Toothpaste

Ingredients:

4 Tablespoons of Bentonite Clay

3-4 Tablespoons Jojoba Oil

10 drops of Peppermint Essential Oil

10 drops of Tea Tree Essential Oil

1 teaspoon of Cinnamon powder

1 teaspoon of Spearmint powder

3-4 drops of Rosemary Extract

Instructions:

Combine the Carrier oil and the Essential oils in a glass jar and mix evenly.

Place all other ingredients into the glass jar with the oil blend.

Mix thoroughly and form a smooth paste.

Apply a small amount of this paste to your toothbrush and brush your teeth.

Rinse your mouth thoroughly with water after brushing your teeth.

Store this toothpaste in an airtight container.

Remedy 2   Sage Herbal Toothpaste

Ingredients:

4 Tablespoons of Bentonite Clay

3-4 Tablespoons Jojoba Oil

10 drops of Peppermint Essential Oil

10 drops of Eucalyptus Essential Oil

1 teaspoon of Sage powder

1 teaspoon of Spearmint powder

3-4 drops of Rosemary Extract

Instructions:

Combine the Carrier oil and the Essential oils in a glass jar and mix evenly.

Place all other ingredients into the glass jar with the oil blend.

Mix thoroughly and form a smooth paste.

Apply a small amount of this paste to your toothbrush and brush your teeth.

Rinse your mouth thoroughly with water after brushing your teeth.

Store this toothpaste in an airtight container.

Remedy 3   Clove Herbal Toothpaste

Ingredients:

4 Tablespoons of Bentonite Clay

3-4 Tablespoons Jojoba Oil

10 drops of Peppermint Essential Oil

10 drops of Thyme Essential Oil

1 teaspoon of Clove powder

1 teaspoon of Spearmint powder

3-4 drops of Rosemary Extract

Instructions:

Combine the Carrier oil and the Essential oils in a glass jar and mix evenly.

Place all other ingredients into the glass jar with the oil blend.

Mix thoroughly and form a smooth paste.

Apply a small amount of this paste to your toothbrush and brush your teeth.

Rinse your mouth thoroughly with water after brushing your teeth.

Store this toothpaste in an airtight container.

Remedy 4   Cinnamon Herbal Mouthwash

***Ingredients*:**

10 drops of Peppermint Essential Oil

10 drops of Cinnamon Essential Oil

1 teaspoon of Sage powder

1 teaspoon of Ginger powder

1 teaspoon of Chamomile powder

1 cup of hot water

***Instructions*:**

Steep the powdered herbs in hot water for 5-10 minutes.

Strain the infusion, and allow it to cool for 15-20 minutes.

Place this infusion and Essential Oils into an airtight container.

Shake well before each use.

Swish around a small amount of this mouthwash in your mouth for 30 seconds.

Spit it out. Do not swallow.

Remedy 5   Ginger Herbal Mouthwash

Ingredients:

10 drops of Peppermint Essential Oil

10 drops of Spearmint Essential Oil

1 teaspoon of Sage powder

1 teaspoon of Ginger powder

1 teaspoon of Lavender powder

1 cup of hot water

Instructions:

Steep the powdered herbs in hot water for 5-10 minutes.

Strain the infusion, and allow it to cool for 15-20 minutes.

Place this infusion and Essential Oils into an airtight container.

Shake well before each use.

Swish around a small amount of this mouthwash in your mouth for 30 seconds.

Spit it out. Do not swallow.

Remedy 6   Fennel Herbal Mouthwash

Ingredients:

10 drops of Peppermint Essential Oil

10 drops of Fennel Essential Oil

1 teaspoon of Sage powder

1 teaspoon of Ginger powder

1 teaspoon of Neem powder

1 cup of hot water

Instructions:

Steep the powdered herbs in hot water for 5-10 minutes.

Strain the infusion, and allow it to cool for 15-20 minutes.

Place this infusion and Essential Oils into an airtight container.

Shake well before each use.

Swish around a small amount of this mouthwash in your mouth for 30 seconds.

Spit it out. Do not swallow.

Remedy 7   Lavender and Marshmallow Root Tea

Ingredients

1 teaspoon of Lavender powder

1 teaspoon of Marshmallow root

1-2 cups of hot water

1 teaspoon of honey (optional)

Instructions

Steep the Lavender powder and the Marshmallow root in hot water for 7-10 minutes.

Strain, add honey (optional), and drink this aromatic tea!

Remedy 8   Ginger Root Tea

Ingredients

1 teaspoon of Ginger root

1 cup of hot water

1 teaspoon of honey (optional)

Instructions:

Steep the Ginger root in hot water for 7-10 minutes.

Strain, add honey (optional), and drink this soothing tea!

Remedy 9   Licorice Root and Ginger Root Tea

Ingredients

1 teaspoon of Licorice root

1 teaspoon of Ginger root

1-2 cups of hot water

1 teaspoon of honey (optional)

Instructions

Steep both herbal roots in hot water for 7-10 minutes.

Strain, add honey (optional), and drink this delightful tea!

Remedy 10 Pineapple Natural Fruit Juice

Ingredients

½ cup of Pineapple (Peeled, cored, and diced)

1 teaspoon of Basil Powder

2 Tablespoons of honey (optional)

1 cup of water

Instructions

Blend the ingredients.

Pour the juice into a glass.

Drink this nourishing juice!

Remedy 11 Uplifting Natural Fruit Juice

Ingredients

½ cup of Grapes (Stemmed)

½ cup of Blueberries

1 teaspoon of Turmeric Powder

2 Tablespoons of honey (optional)

1-2 cups of water

Instructions

Blend the ingredients.

Pour the juice into a glass.

Drink this sparkling juice!

Remedy 12 Tasty Natural Fruit Juice

Ingredients

½ cup of Apple (Cored and sliced)

½ cup of Kiwi (Peeled and sliced)

1 teaspoon of Catnip Powder

2 Tablespoons of honey (optional)

1-2 cups of water

Instructions

Blend the ingredients.

Pour the juice into a glass.

Drink this reviving juice!

- **Bonus Tips:** maintain proper oral hygiene practices; remember to have a healthy diet.

CANKER SORES

Remedy 1   Neem Herbal Toothpaste

Ingredients:

4 Tablespoons of Bentonite Clay

3-4 Tablespoons Jojoba Oil

10 drops of Peppermint Essential Oil

10 drops of Oregano Essential Oil

1 teaspoon of Neem powder

1 teaspoon of Spearmint powder

3-4 drops of Rosemary Extract

Instructions:

Combine the Carrier oil and the Essential oils in a glass jar and mix evenly.

Place all other ingredients into the glass jar with the oil blend.

Mix thoroughly and form a smooth paste.

Apply a small amount of this paste to your toothbrush and brush your teeth.

Rinse your mouth thoroughly with water after brushing your teeth.

Store this toothpaste in an airtight container.

Remedy 2   Goldenseal Herbal Toothpaste

Ingredients:

4 Tablespoons of Bentonite Clay

3-4 Tablespoons Jojoba Oil

10 drops of Peppermint Essential Oil

10 drops of Wintergreen Essential Oil

1 teaspoon of Goldenseal powder

1 teaspoon of Spearmint powder

3-4 drops of Rosemary Extract

Instructions:

Combine the Carrier oil and the Essential oils in a glass jar and mix evenly.

Place all other ingredients into the glass jar with the oil blend.

Mix thoroughly and form a smooth paste.

Apply a small amount of this paste to your toothbrush and brush your teeth.

Rinse your mouth thoroughly with water after brushing your teeth.

Store this toothpaste in an airtight container.

Remedy 3   Basil Herbal Toothpaste

Ingredients:

4 Tablespoons of Bentonite Clay

3-4 Tablespoons Jojoba Oil

10 drops of Peppermint Essential Oil

10 drops of Basil Essential Oil

1 teaspoon of Slippery Elm powder

1 teaspoon of Spearmint powder

3-4 drops of Rosemary Extract (preservative)

Instructions:

Combine the Carrier oil and the Essential oils in a glass jar and mix evenly.

Place all other ingredients into the glass jar with the oil blend.

Mix thoroughly and form a smooth paste.

Apply a small amount of this paste to your toothbrush and brush your teeth.

Rinse your mouth thoroughly with water after brushing your teeth.

Store this toothpaste in an airtight container.

Remedy 4   Lemongrass Herbal Mouthwash

***Ingredients*:**

10 drops of Peppermint Essential Oil

10 drops of Lemongrass Essential Oil

1 teaspoon of Sage powder

1 teaspoon of Ginger powder

1 teaspoon of Lemon Balm powder

1 cup of hot water

***Instructions*:**

Steep the powdered herbs in hot water for 5-10 minutes.

Strain the infusion, and allow it to cool for 15-20 minutes.

Place this infusion and Essential Oils into an airtight container.

Shake well before each use.

Swish around a small amount of this mouthwash in your mouth for 30 seconds.

Spit it out. Do not swallow.

Remedy 5   Peppermint Herbal Mouthwash

Ingredients:

10 drops of Peppermint Essential Oil

10 drops of Tea Tree Essential Oil

1 teaspoon of Sage powder

1 teaspoon of Ginger powder

1 teaspoon of Licorice powder

1 cup of hot water

Instructions:

Steep the powdered herbs in hot water for 5-10 minutes.

Strain the infusion, and allow it to cool for 15-20 minutes.

Place this infusion and Essential Oils into an airtight container.

Shake well before each use.

Swish around a small amount of this mouthwash in your mouth for 30 seconds.

Spit it out. Do not swallow.

Remedy 6   Frankincense Herbal Mouthwash

***Ingredients*:**

10 drops of Peppermint Essential Oil

10 drops of Frankincense Essential Oil

1 teaspoon of Sage powder

1 teaspoon of Ginger powder

1 teaspoon of White Willow Bark powder

1 cup of hot water

Instructions:

Steep the powdered herbs in hot water for 5-10 minutes.

Strain the infusion, and allow it to cool for 15-20 minutes.

Place this infusion and Essential Oils into an airtight container.

Shake well before each use.

Swish around a small amount of this mouthwash in your mouth for 30 seconds.

Spit it out. Do not swallow.

Remedy 7   Green Tea and Yellow Dock Root Tea

Ingredients

1 teaspoon of Green Tea powder

1 teaspoon of Yellow Dock root

1-2 cups of hot water

1 teaspoon of honey (optional)

Instructions

Steep the Green Tea powder and the Yellow Dock root in hot water for 7-10 minutes.

Strain, add honey (optional), and drink this aromatic tea!

Remedy 8   Comfrey Root Tea

Ingredients

1 teaspoon of Comfrey root

1 cup of hot water

1 teaspoon of honey (optional)

Instructions:

Steep the Comfrey root in hot water for 7-10 minutes.

Strain, add honey (optional), and drink this soothing tea!

Remedy 9 Echinacea Root and Valerian Root Tea

Ingredients

1 teaspoon of Echinacea root

1 teaspoon of Valerian root

1-2 cups of hot water

1 teaspoon of honey (optional)

Instructions

Steep both herbal roots in hot water for 7-10 minutes.

Strain, add honey (optional), and drink this delightful tea!

Remedy 10 Watermelon Natural Fruit Juice

Ingredients

½ cup of Watermelon (Diced and seeded)

1 teaspoon of Red Clover Powder

2 Tablespoons of honey (optional)

1 cup of water

Instructions

Blend the ingredients.

Pour the juice into a glass.

Drink this nourishing juice!

Remedy 11 Berry-Blast Natural Fruit Juice

Ingredients

½ cup of Blackberries

½ cup of Blueberries

1 teaspoon of Ginseng Powder

2 Tablespoons of honey (optional)

1-2 cups of water

Instructions

Blend the ingredients.

Pour the juice into a glass.

Drink this sparkling juice!

Remedy 12 Berry-Crave Natural Fruit Juice

Ingredients

½ cup of Cranberries

½ cup of Strawberries (Hulled and sliced)

1 teaspoon of Lemon Verbena Powder

2 Tablespoons of honey (optional)

1-2 cups of water

Instructions

Blend the ingredients.

Pour the juice into a glass.

Drink this reviving juice!

- **Bonus Tips:** maintain proper oral hygiene; remember to have a healthy diet.

CONCLUSION

144 Herbal Remedies For Natural Healing is a book designed to help guide you in using simple natural remedies to treat illnesses and alleviate their symptoms. We hope that as you read, you will benefit greatly from the general knowledge shared in this book.

We have more books on the way and we ask for your continued support as we bring helpful and informative knowledge in this time of **climatic changes.** May our Heavenly Father Yahweh Elohiym and our Savior, Yahshua Ha Mashiach guide you on this journey to long life.

Visit me at:

My Herbal Products Store

eliyahmashiachherbalstore.com

All My Books

https://www.amazon.com/author/eliyahmashiach

My Email

eliyahmashiach@gmail.com

My Tiktok

https://www.tiktok.com/@eliyahmashiach2

My Instagram @eliyahmashiach_

Thank you for all the support and love family.

Notes Pages

Made in the USA
Las Vegas, NV
07 May 2024